Seeing

Is

Believing

Enhancing Your Vision

John P. Frangie, M.D.

Seeing Is Believing: Enhancing Your Vision
Copyright © 2012 by John P. Frangie, M.D.

ISBN 978-0-9848956-0-1

Dedication

This monogram is dedicated to our staff members who unfailingly work to provide the data necessary to take care of our patients. These people work hard every day and are not recognized nearly enough. While I may sometimes forget to express my gratitude, I am always aware that one cannot deliver a meaningful experience to the patient without the diligence and kindness these men and women consistently demonstrate.

Table of Contents

Preface

One of my most enduring childhood birthday presents was given to me at age eleven by my parents. The gift was a booklet with the poem "If" by Rudyard Kipling. I know my understanding of the writing was limited at age eleven (indeed, some 40 years later, I still question some of my interpretations), but I don't think Mr. Kipling would be opposed to a sixth grader extracting his own interpretations (even if it was not precisely that of the author). One verse, in particular, I later used to guide my patient interactions:

If you can talk with crowds and keep your virtue,
Or walk with Kings—nor lose the common touch,

I apply this to my practice by remembering that patients are not (usually) optical engineers, but this does not diminish their desire to know what's going on with their eyes and what needs to be done to fix it. The purpose of this text is not to be a condescending "dumbed down" treatise about your visual sense, but rather a practical discussion on how one's eyes work, why the system fails and what remedies are available. Some parts will be painfully basic and intuitive, others more scientific and appropriate for those optics aficionados who mistakenly picked up this book expecting a dissertation on Fourier Analysis, or some other optical esoterica. If you are a patient and I have already spoken to you about cataracts, you will undoubtedly be familiar with some of the terms and analogies in this book.

Visual aids play a significant role in teaching both physicians and patients. This book has a number of figures which hopefully will help clarify information. In addition, I have taken advantage of the Internet, and will occasionally refer you to videos/animations available on my website at www.frangieeye.com .

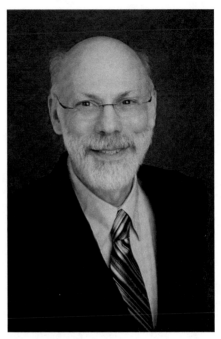

Michael S. Feinberg, O.D.

Foreword

I first became aware of Dr. John Frangie in 1989 at
a seminar he gave for other doctors at the Boston
University Medical School while he was in his
second year of residency. He spoke about the
cornea as it is affected by disease and dystrophy. I
was impressed by the depth of his knowledge and
the care he took in his presentation. Every question
asked was an opportunity for further explanation.

Over the years, he has established a level of care that serves as an example of what proper surgical eye care should be.

Before surgery is performed, the patient should know what the procedure is, why it is necessary and what to expect as a result of it. This book provides the patient with enough information to give his or her informed consent for the procedures discussed. Topics that can be difficult and complicated are explained in understandable words.

From reading this book, it is clear that Dr. Frangie still retains a sense of joy and wonder with regards to his chosen profession, which then makes each and every one of his surgeries a work of art and science.

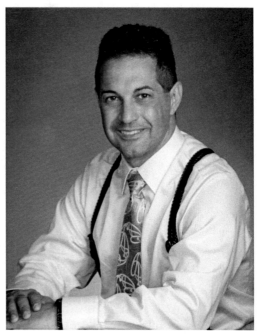

John P. Frangie, M.D.

Introduction

Cataract surgery is among the most commonly performed and successful procedures in the world. The procedure is typically performed under a local anesthetic, facilitating patient acceptance and rapid recovery.

Despite the overwhelming popularity of the surgery and the typically excellent results it offers, there are a number of common misgivings shared by potential patients. While it is understandable that patients may not comprehend the nuances of the procedure, many individuals have little concept of what a cataract actually is, or how it affects one's vision, and subsequently, lifestyle.

It is my hope that this book will serve as a teaching instrument for my patients and their families, as the informed patient is better able to play a role in helping me deliver successful ophthalmic care.

Chapter One

How the Eye Works

The eye is a "sensory organ," that is, it takes in physical impulses (photons of light) and converts them into electrical impulses which are interpreted in the brain in order to orient its "beholder." The simplicity of the eye's optics is matched by the elegance of its microstructure.

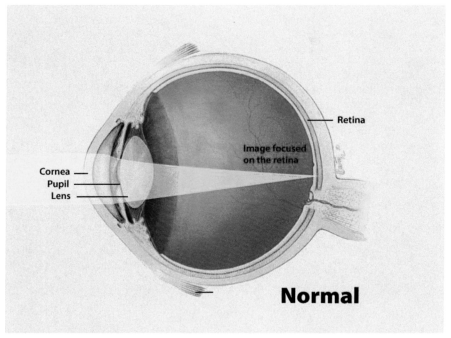

Cornea
Pupil
Lens
Retina
Image focused on the retina
Normal

Courtesy of National Eye Institute, National Institute of Health
Figure 1 Cross-section view of the eye

To simplify, the eye is very much like a camera. Light enters the front of the eye (Figure 1) as a broad beam, and is focused to a tiny pinpoint in the back of the eye. The first structure that bends or "focuses" light is the **cornea**. The cornea is the clear outer window upon which a patient's contact lenses rest. Light then passes through the **pupil**, the dark circle we see when we look directly at each other's eyes. The pupil is the equivalent of a camera diaphragm, and is located in the center of the **iris** – the part of the eye which has the eye "color."

The **lens** is the second and final light-bending structure. The lens is located just behind the pupil, and possesses about one third of the eye's light-bending, or **refractive** strength. In the ideal or "perfect" eye, after being focused by the lens, the light rays emanating from an image will be focused upon the **retina**, which is the "film" of our camera.

Once the image rays fall upon the retina, photoreceptors are triggered, which cause an electrical impulse to be generated. These impulses are propagated to the **optic nerve** and travel to the brain where they are interpreted as sight. Hence the correct answer to the trick question occasionally posed during physiology examinations -"With which of the body's organs do we see?"-is "The brain."

Chapter Two

What is a Cataract?

When I ask patients if they know what a cataract is, many will respond, "Why yes, Doctor, many of my friends have had their cataracts removed. A cataract is a skin (or film) that grows across the surface of the eye."

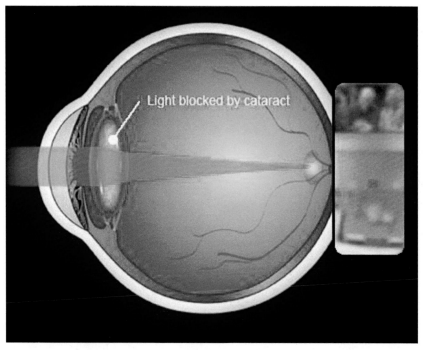

Courtesy of Bausch & Lomb Company

Figure 2 Cataract causing vision to be blurry

Actually, a **cataract** is not a skin or abnormal growth on the surface of the eye, but rather a change in one of the eye's internal components, the **lens.** As you now know, the lens is the second light-bending structure in the eye. The term cataract describes when the lens loses its transparency,

(Figure 2) thereby preventing the focusing of light rays efficiently upon the retina and ultimately causing the eye to generate a compromised or blurred image.

The lens has four primary components. The **zonules** suspend the lens from the **ciliary muscle**. This connection between the lens and the circular ciliary muscle allow the young, flexible lens to change its shape, and hence how much it bends light. The flexible lens (which is the disposition of our natural lens, until approximately the age of forty) is able to change its focusing strength and therefore we are able to focus light rays from images that are both near and distant. The ability to focus clearly upon images at different distances is known as **accommodation**. As mentioned, we lose our ability to accommodate around the age of 40, and it deteriorates gradually until virtually all accommodative function is lost at around 65 years of age. This gradual loss of lens flexibility accounts for the need for progressively stronger reading glasses between the ages of 40 and 65 years.

The zonules connect to the **capsular bag** or capsule (or "**the bag**" as it is referred to by surgeons). The capsule is a thin, clear envelope which surrounds the inner, light-bending (or refracting) tissues of the lens. The lens has two primary zones: the inner **nucleus** and the surrounding outer **cortex**. The outer cortex has many layers which surround and come in contact with the more uniform, "disc-shaped" central nucleus. The cortex tends to be less dense, and softer than the nucleus.

There are a number of different types of cataracts. The cataract type is typically classified by where in the lens the specific abnormality occurs; alternatively, cataracts may be characterized by the condition which caused the loss of lens transparency. Occasionally, certain types of cataracts pose special demands upon the surgeon as they tend to be associated with conditions that make the removal of the cataract more challenging (for instance, posterior polar cataracts and traumatic cataracts).

Chapter Three

A Recent History of Cataract Surgery

Cataract surgery in its most basic form has been practiced for centuries; indeed, the ancient Greeks described a procedure to restore vision loss caused by cataract formation. For the purposes of this discussion, we will concentrate on the changes brought to us in the past half century. Interestingly, the recent history of cataract surgery has evolved as intraocular lens technology has evolved.

The intraocular lens is the synthetic replacement lens which is implanted after the removal of the cataract. The use of an **intraocular lens**, or **implant,** did not gain momentum until the last two decades of the twentieth century. Prior to the use of implants, ophthalmologists performed a cataract procedure known as an **intracapsular cataract extraction (ICCE)**. In this case, the cataract was removed in its entirety, including its protective envelope (the capsule). The early days of ICCE predated the use of operating microscopes, so surgeons were relegated to using surgical loupes, specialized spectacles which provided magnification.

The limitations of the loupes dictated that surgeons use relatively thick-gauge suture material. The suture material was silk – a fine material for clothing, but nonetheless irritating when used to stitch a large surgical wound on the ocular surface.

Additionally, the relatively low magnification provided by the loupes often resulted in a less-than-perfect matching of the layers of the surgical wound.

The lack of an intraocular lens (IOL), meant that the function of the lens (which was removed because it was cataractous) needed to be compensated for either by full-time use of a contact lens or by significantly enhancing the strength of the patient's glasses. These "cataract glasses," also known as **aphakic** (meaning lens-less) spectacles were very thick and were characterized by lenses which had the shape of a fried egg. Due to the strength of these lenses, there were numerous optical aberrations which caused significant distortion of images – but these glasses did provide a degree of functional vision.

In the latter half of the twentieth century, ophthalmologists discovered that by preserving the lens capsule at the time of surgery, this structure could be utilized to support an intraocular lens. The optical strength of the IOL replaced that of the surgically removed lens; therefore, patients were no longer encumbered by their dependency upon contact lenses or heavy aphakic spectacles. Not only was an intraocular lens more convenient, but the quality of vision was enhanced. This form of surgery, which maintained the natural envelope of the cataract, was termed **extracapsular cataract surgery (ECCE),** and you can see the video of it at www.frangieeye.com

The first instances of extracapsular cataract surgery called upon the surgeon to remove the dense, inner nucleus portion of the cataract in one single step. The relatively large size of the nucleus required a large incision, extending about 160 degrees around the perimeter of the cornea. Accordingly, the surgeon had to sew the incision closed after placement of the intraocular lens.

The next significant advancement of ECCE was the ability to gently disassemble the cataract inside the eye. The micro-instrumentation used to remove the cataract with this technique only required an incision of a few millimeters. This type of cataract procedure still preserved the lens capsule, and therefore was still an extracapsular procedure. The process of breaking the lens into small particles within the eye was called **phacoemulsification.** The wound still had to be opened to allow placement of the IOL, but this problem would eventually be solved with the advent of foldable intraocular lenses.

Chapter Four

What is an Intraocular Lens?

Strictly speaking, an intraocular lens (IOL) is an artificial lens which is placed within the eye. For years, the term intraocular lens exclusively referred to lenses that were placed in the eye following removal of a cataract. In recent years, a specialized subclass of intraocular lenses known as **phakic** lenses has been introduced. These lenses are placed in eyes that are healthy and have not developed cataracts in an attempt to decrease the patient's need for contact lenses and glasses (the implantable contact lens is discussed in chapter 11: Other Surgical Methods of Vision Correction). For the purpose of this chapter, the term "intraocular lens" will refer to those lenses placed following removal of a cataract. Another commonly used term for IOL is **lens implant**.

The improved visual function offered by implants revolutionized cataract surgery. Following World War II, Sir Harold Ridley developed the first intraocular lenses. Ridley examined fighter pilots and found it interesting that some of these pilots had shards of the canopies from British Spitfire fighter planes embedded in their eyes. The canopy fragments did not appear to cause scarring or inflammation, so Ridley surmised that the same material would be well-tolerated if used as a surgical implant. The fighter canopies were constructed from Plexiglass, also known as polymethylmethacrylate (PMMA). While the PMMA compound did indeed prove to be well tolerated, it took years of different designs and processing techniques to create an IOL that was both well tolerated and gentle to the delicate surrounding ocular tissues.

Typically, in modern cataract surgery, the IOL will be positioned in the capsular bag. The lenses which are placed "in the bag" have two components. (Figure 3)

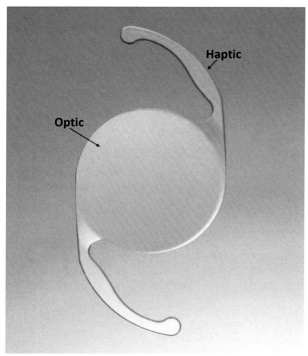

Courtesy of Alcon Laboratories

Figure 3   Intraocular Lens (IOL)

The central round portion of the lens is the part of the lens with the optical strength; this structure is called the **optic**. The optic has two supporting "arms" positioned 180 degrees away from each other. The supporting arms are referred to as **haptics**. The haptics are essentially two flexible struts which spread out equally to the edges of the bag. The optic is maintained in the middle of the bag, and is passively supported by the haptics, and hence no sutures (stitches) are required for support. As time passes, the capsular bag "shrink wraps" around the IOL, further stabilizing its position in the eye.

Phacoemulsification, (see video available at www.frangieeye.com) is the operation characterized by the disassembly of the cataract nucleus inside the eye and results in an external incision which requires only a few stitches to close. The decrease in external wound size initiated the trend toward modern small-incision, "no-stitch" surgery. However, while the process of *removing* the cataract no longer required a large incision, the implants still had 6.0 -7.0mm rigid PMMA optics (that's right, we were still using Plexiglass routinely as an implant material in the 1980s!). Therefore, the 3-4mm phacoemulsification incision still had to be extended significantly, in order to implant the IOL.

Polymer chemistry in the late 1980s provided the impetus for the next significant breakthrough in cataract surgery. The introduction of silicone and acrylic materials that were soft, gave surgeons the ability to *fold* the implants in order to keep the incision small. Once in the eye, the IOL would unfold in the bag, assuming its normal, full state. The latest lens delivery systems involve loading these lenses into a round cartridge and injecting the implant into the eye, where it slowly unfolds and assumes its normal shape.

In summary, the evolution of cataract surgery has mirrored our progress in lens development. These devices have evolved from roughly machined pieces of Plexiglass to pliable, UV-blocking polymer composites that allow implantation through incisions of less than 2 millimeters. Incisions that are small, stable and watertight allow patients to rapidly achieve their maximal vision while limiting recovery time.

Recently, IOLs have made another quantum leap with significant improvements in the enhanced visual function they offer patients. These advanced technology lenses still allow surgeons to create microscopic incisions, and patients still experience the benefit of a very limited convalescence. Now they can offer patients crisper and greater visual function than most have had in decades.

Chapter Five

Presbyopic Implants

Having been a refractive surgeon for more than two decades, I have had the occasion to treat thousands of patients who wished to realize the dream of having their eyes function "normally." When I delve further, the motivation understandably varies on a case-by-case basis: a young woman wants to enter military service, an older patient is concerned that his eyes are affecting his ability to react while driving at night, a young mother is worried that she won't be able to find her glasses in the middle of the night should her child need her urgently, or a man simply wants "to be able to wake up and see things clearly." Despite the numerous legitimate reasons for seeking help with their eyes, most patients' definition of seeing normally is to be able to function fully and effectively with no or only minimal dependence on a **prosthesis** (glasses or contact lenses).

Modern cataract surgery allows the surgeon to not only correct the blurriness and loss of acuity that occurs with a cataract, but also to improve other conditions-**nearsightedness, farsightedness, astigmatism** and **presbyopia**. Nearsightedness occurs when the eye's ability to see close (or near) objects is better than its ability to see objects in the distance. Conversely, farsightedness is the condition when an eye is able to see distant objects clearer than close objects. Farsightedness is often confused with presbyopia, though presbyopia is actually the eye's *age-related* loss of clarity for near objects. Almost universally, presbyopia affects patients in their forties; indeed, the term presbyopia is derived from the Greek language meaning "aging eye." Astigmatism is a term which usually relates to the curvature of the eye's outer window, the cornea. Astigmatism will be described in more detail in chapter 7: Astigmatism-Correcting Intraocular Lenses.

Presbyopia is one of the most frustrating conditions that plague patients, and because it is age-related, it is virtually universal. The ability for the youthful eye to clearly see objects at distance and moments later just inches away from the face is a function of the natural lens being able to change its shape, a process termed **accommodation**. The accommodative response involves a muscular process.

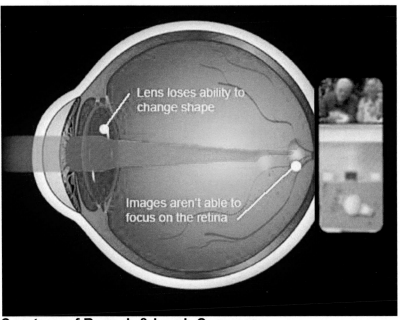

Figure 4 Presbyopia

The lens capsule is attached to zonules which in turn are connected to the ring-shaped **ciliary muscle**. Contraction of the ciliary muscle *releases* tension on the zonules which in turn relax their pull upon the lens. The lens then assumes a more spherical shape, and bends light to a greater degree (delivering more **optical power**). The additional power allows the eye to see closer objects. Therefore the optically "normal" eye which can see things clearly without correction at distance, also has the ability to *adjust its focus* so near objects may also be seen clearly without correction. The lens loses its ability to become spherical (or adjust its focus) beginning around the age of forty (Figure 4), and in so doing it begins to lose the ability to provide the extra optical power to see near objects. Therefore, in order for that forty-something year-old patient to see the near objects as clearly as she could a few short years earlier, we have to artificially replace that optical power which the eye has lost– enter reading glasses.

The surgeon is able to correct nearsightedness and farsightedness by adjusting the **intraocular lens power**. Remember the discussion regarding the structures of the eye? There are two light-bending or refracting elements, the cornea and the lens. As you know, a cataract is when the lens loses its transparency, so in order to re-establish a clear path for light to travel; the cataract is removed from the eye. The natural lens of the eye bends light to a certain degree, and that particular amount of light-bending capacity is the power of that lens. If the surgeon removed the cataract of a nearsighted patient, and replaced the cataract with an implant which had the same power as the cataractous lens, the patient would still be nearsighted after their surgery. Similarly, if the surgeon was operating on the cataract of a farsighted patient and placed an IOL which had the same power as the patient's natural lens, that patient would still be farsighted after his surgery.

Now here is the neat part for those patients who could not see clearly for most of their lives without glasses or contacts because they were either nearsighted or farsighted. Through the use of a series of measurements, your surgeon is able to essentially incorporate the power of the eyeglass lens or contact lens you wore before surgery into the IOL. The integration of the eye's correction into the implant leaves the eye with a greatly reduced need for correction after surgery. However, unless a specialized implant was used, the eye is still presbyopic! That is, the traditional single focus (also known as monofocal) implant may allow the eye to see clearly at a given distance, but there is no ability to focus at more than one distance, so one particular distance is in focus while all other points in front and beyond that one distance are anywhere from slightly to significantly out-of-focus.

The only way that an eye with a monofocal intraocular lenses can focus clearly at more than one distance is by the external placement of lenses that have different focal lengths or distances – **bifocal** (*two* focal distances) spectacles, **trifocal** (*three* focal distances) or **progressive** spectacles (theoretically many different focal points depending upon where the pupil is in relation to the spectacle lens).

The next significant breakthrough in cataract surgery came with the introduction of **presbyopic intraocular lenses.** Presbyopic IOLs offer patients the opportunity to again focus clearly on objects at different distances without the use of spectacles. Implanting the advanced technology presbyopic lenses gives surgeons the ability to correct numerous different optical aberrations – nearsightedness, farsightedness, astigmatism and **presbyopia**--thereby restoring the eye's focusing ability which had been lost as a function of aging. There are two primary ways which presbyopic (or advanced technology) lenses work. The first type of presbyopic lens offered in the United States was the accommodating intraocular lens. (Figures 5 A & 5 B) This lens is built on a flexible platform.

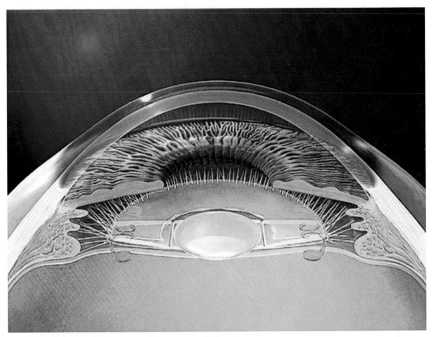

Courtesy of Bausch & Lomb Company

Figure 5 A The Crystalens moves forward with muscle contraction, enhancing near vision.

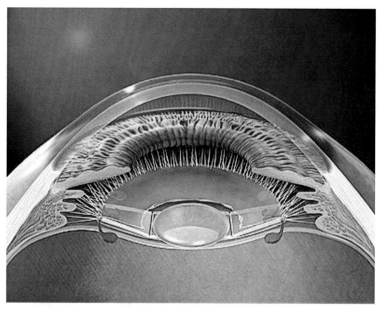

Figure 5 B The Crystalens sitting in "relaxed" position focuses distant objects.

The accommodating style IOLs are actually able to flex in response to the ciliary muscle contracting – in a manner similar to how a natural lens would change shape in the younger eye. Very slight motion and flexing of the lens allows the eye to gain more "power" when a patient focuses from distant to near objects.(Figure 5 A & 5 B)

A video of Crystalens implantation may be viewed at www.frangieeye.com.

The other mechanism by which an intraocular lens may replace the loss of accommodation is through multifocal optics. The multifocal system has a modified optic (lens portion of the IOL) which is able to modify the light entering the eye and focus some light for near visualization and another portion focuses the energy to allow visualization of distant images. Simply speaking, the multifocal implants, apportions the light to different focal lengths so different distances are in focus; this occurs without effort from the patient and is a totally passive system. Thus, patients do not have to worry about looking through a certain portion of their implant to see at a specific distance.

In summary, advances in cataract surgery and its outcomes have gone hand-in-hand with the evolution of intraocular lenses. The latest quantum leap in IOL technology is the introduction of presbyopic intraocular lenses. Unlike standard monofocal IOLs, these lenses restore the eye's ability to have a range of clear vision.

"So Doctor," you say, **"It is so nice that you know about these new implants, but which one do I choose?"**

This indeed is the operative question, and the answer is one you will often hear in medicine: **"It depends!"** The first issue to determine is whether the health of your eye will allow you to benefit from this new technology. The medical criteria are discussed in the next chapter.

Chapter Six

Am I a Candidate for the Advanced Technology Intraocular Lens?

While most people would select the enhanced optical performance offered by the presbyopic lenses, these implants are not appropriate for all patients. There are a number of conditions and diseases which either decrease or totally neutralize the benefits these lenses can deliver. While many of these limitations are agreed upon by most cataract specialists, there may be room for debate among surgeons, so I will offer you my own guidelines (and preferences) based upon the specific ocular condition. Of course, I have a discussion with each patient who has any of these conditions and is considering optimizing his/her cataract procedure with an advanced technology IOL. Accordingly, these patients realize that their eyes are not 100% typical, and there is the very real possibility that the eyes will not see 20/20 after ANY type of IOL is implanted.

Macular Degeneration

Age-related macular degeneration (ARMD) is the subject of numerous articles, chapters and indeed textbooks. To attempt to describe it in any detail is well beyond the scope of this text. Suffice it to say that macular degeneration is typically an age-related loss of the cells which comprise the retina – the "film" where images are generated in your eye.

While there are a few dissenting opinions at the time this monolog is being printed, most surgeons queried will not recommend the use of multifocal IOLs in patients with moderate to severe macular degeneration. It is typically my custom NOT to implant multifocal presbyopic IOLs in eyes that have macular degeneration. The disease typically is progressive (that is, it gets worse as time passes) so it is questionable if a patient would appreciate any benefit with these lenses. In contrast, I have had success implanting accommodating intraocular lenses (the lenses which flex like our natural lens) in patients with early to moderate macular degeneration. Macular degeneration tends not to affect the performance of the accommodating IOLs – presumably due to their more physiologic mechanism of action.

Severe Dry Eye Syndrome

The cornea is the outer "window" and primary light-bending structure of the eye. The cornea is covered by a thin layer of tears, the **precorneal tear film** (PCTF). The tear film protects the eye from dust, allergens and infectious agents, as well as serving as an avenue for the immune system. Additionally, a stable, contiguous PCTF is vital for the cornea to fulfill its function as the eye's primary focusing element.

Dry eye syndrome is the condition when the surface of the eye has a deficient or unstable PCTF. As a result, there are "dry spots" on the surface of the cornea. The dry spots can cause irritation to the extent that the patient experiences excessive tearing – this is caused by the dryness becoming a noxious stimulus which causes a physiologic response similar to the tearing that occurs when there is a piece of sand or dust in the eye. The excessive tear volume actually causes the vision to decrease, in addition to introducing the inconvenience of having tears running down one's cheek in severe cases.

The patient's vision may also be affected even when there is not any discomfort or excessive tearing. The dryness may cause an irregularity upon the surface of the cornea which results in light scattering. The process of light scattering introduces a source of inefficiency in the eye's optical system. A cornea that scatters light is described by ophthalmologists as having **aberrations**. Aberrations are imperfections which cause light to defocus, resulting in a blurring of images, as light does not pass efficiently to the retina. Highly aberrated corneas prevent ALL IOLs from working optimally, but especially **multifocal presbyopic** lenses from working effectively. For this reason, I do not recommend placing multifocal intraocular lenses in eyes with severe dry eye.

In contrast, accommodating presbyopic lenses and astigmatism-correcting lenses may be placed in eyes with significant corneal optical aberrations; while the results may not be "perfect" 20/20 vision, the results of cataract surgery in patients with aberrated corneas can be quite gratifying.

Dry eye syndrome is not the only condition which results in cornea-based optical aberrations. **Corneal scarring** from disease or trauma may introduce optical aberrations. **Radial keratotomy** was a popular refractive surgery procedure in the 1980s and 90s. The keratotomy incisions induce optical aberrations, and actually induce multifocality of the cornea. Accordingly, most cornea specialists will not place a multifocal IOL in an eye that has had radial keratotomy. Instead, the use of the accommodating presbyopic IOL in "post-RK" eyes has resulted in some excellent outcomes as these patients enjoy the dual benefit of a **multifocal cornea** combined with an accommodating IOL.

The decision on whether to implant a presbyopic lens (or indeed perform cataract surgery at all!) in a patient with dry eye, or any eye that has corneal disease can be difficult. Among the factors to be considered preoperatively include the degree of dryness, cause of dryness, degree of visual debilitation, visual potential of the eye and patient expectations.

Diabetes Mellitus

The ocular sequelae of diabetes mellitus were among the leading causes of blindness in the United States in the mid to late 1900s. Diabetes affects virtually all of the body's systems and the eye is no exception. Cornea, lens and retina are all potential targets of this disease. Diabetic retinopathy, like macular degeneration, is a disease which has been well chronicled, and an extensive discussion about diabetic ocular disease is beyond the scope of this text.

The process of **diabetic retinopathy** is caused by serum glucose compromising the competence of the vascular endothelium. That is, abnormally high levels of blood sugar cause blood vessels to leak into the retina, causing a loss of retinal function – again a process where the "film" of the camera is impaired. I generally do not recommend the multifocal presbyopic intraocular lenses in cases where the patient's retinal function has been affected (although the accommodating lenses may be considered).

There is one diabetic condition where I typically do NOT recommend either type of presbyopic intraocular lens; the condition is called **proliferative diabetic retinopathy**. In proliferative retinopathy, the serum glucose has so adversely affected the retinal vasculature that there is a gross lack of oxygen being delivered to the retina. This lack of oxygen, or **hypoxia**, results in the growth of new *abnormal* retina vessels which have a tendency to actually bleed inside the eye. Eyes that have this degree of impairment from diabetes do not typically realize a significant benefit from presbyopic IOLs.

Chapter Seven

Astigmatism-Correcting Intraocular Lenses

Chapter one described some basics of ophthalmic optics. The front of the eye serves as a focusing element to bring a sharp image upon the retina. Creating a sharp retinal image requires that the cornea and lens each create a single focal point. (Figure 6 A)

Figure 6 A Eye with normal cornea

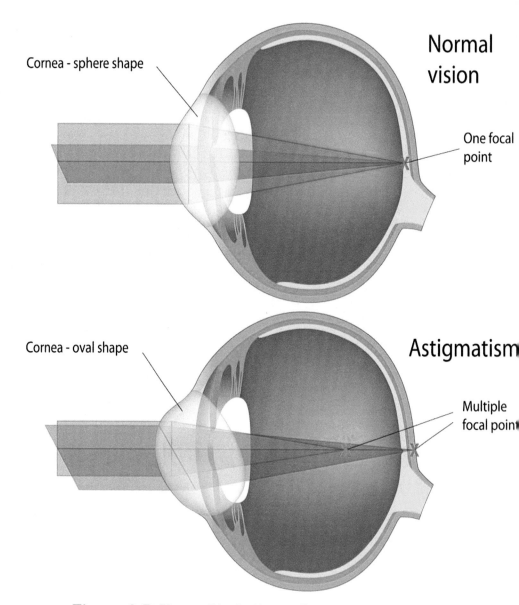

Cornea - sphere shape

Normal vision

One focal point

Cornea - oval shape

Astigmatism

Multiple focal point

Figure 6 B Eye with Astigmatism cornea.

Generating a single focal point for the cornea requires that the cornea has a round "dome" shape with the same degree of curvature for 360 degrees, therefore no matter what place light enters the cornea, it is bent to the same degree en route to the lens. Astigmatism, specifically *corneal astigmatism*, may be described as the condition where the cornea has at least two radii of curvature. Less technically explained, the outer window of the eye has a more oval or "football" shape (Figure 6 B) The two different curvatures of the cornea generate two different focal points because light rays are bent differently depending upon which part of the cornea they enter; as a result even a perfectly symmetric crystalline lens or standard IOL will not be able to bring the light rays to a single retinal focal point, so the eye does not create a clear image for the patient.

Before the advent of advanced technology implants, removing the cataract involved exclusively removing and replacing the eye's lens and if an eye had significant corneal astigmatism before cataract surgery, the condition would exist after surgery. The introduction of **astigmatism-correcting** or **toric** intraocular lenses finally gave astigmatic patients an answer to correct their vision, not only reversing the effects of the cataract, but actually making their uncorrected vision *better* than it had been for years – typically decades! Toric lenses correct vision in a manner that standard single focus lenses cannot – the toric lens, like the astigmatic eye's cornea, also has two curvatures. Toric lenses are placed precisely in relation to the eye's particular corneal curvature so that the toricity of the IOL neutralizes the patient's corneal astigmatism.

Correcting or "neutralizing" the corneal astigmatism creates a more precise focal image, thereby reducing or totally eliminating the cornea-induced blur (in "ophthalmology speak" this is called "collapsing the Conoid of Sturm," or reducing the distance between the two corneal focal points. Please note: stating this at parties or other social events will not win you acclaim, and will quite likely result in your prompt removal).

Chapter Eight

Your Cataract Treatment

Modern cataract surgery is a "day stay" procedure. Most **ambulatory surgicenters** (ASCs) and hospitals allow the patient to remain in their clothes and merely wear a gown, cap and shoe covers in the operating room. Typically, patients are allowed to have a light breakfast. On the day of treatment, you will be at the hospital or ASC for about three hours. The procedure is usually performed under topical anesthesia, which means drops are applied to the eye for comfort, in addition to dilating drops. The dilating drops increase the size of the pupil so the surgeon has easier access to the cataract. In addition, an intravenous catheter is placed to facilitate the use of sedation during your procedure.

You will then be brought into the treatment room, where the anesthesiologist and circulating nurse will make sure you are comfortable and well-positioned for your procedure. Once you are positioned appropriately, the next member of our surgical team, the scrub nurse, will use an antiseptic solution to "prep" your eye. The scrub nurse will then place a light drape around your eye so that there will be a sterile **surgical field**. Alas! We can get to the actual process of removing the cataract and restoring your vision. (A video of this is available at www.frangieeye.com.)

The surgical microscope will then be positioned about one foot above the operative eye. The microscope has intense lighting and in combination with the dilation, the brightness can be very impressive. The light intensity is notable only for a few moments, after which your eye will adapt to the brightness. The surgeon then places a small eyelid supporting instrument so that you will not have to worry about blinking.

Utilizing the microscope to magnify your eye, the surgeon creates a small peripheral corneal incision that allows controlled access to the internal structures of the eye. The surgeon has micro instruments which enable him/her to address the cataract through the pupil. The next step involves creating a small opening in the cataract capsule. This opening is about 5 millimeters in diameter, and it is through this opening the surgeon applies ultrasonic energy to gently disassemble the cataract nucleus into tiny fragments. The cataract fragments are suspended in the balanced saline solution which the surgeon gently rinses from your eye.

Once the nucleus has been removed, the cortex of the cataract remains. As the cortex is typically very soft, no energy is needed to disassemble it, and cortical removal is usually performed with a very low power vacuum delivered by an instrument called the irrigation/aspiration hand piece. Cortical clean-up completes the process of cataract extraction, and the eye is now ready for intraocular lens implantation.

As described earlier, today's IOLs are made of very soft, flexible polymers, so they can be folded in order to be placed through the very small corneal incision directly into the capsular bag. The lens then unfolds in a very slow, controlled fashion inside "the bag" and thereby occupies the location of the natural lens it replaced. The lens is supported in the capsule by the flexible haptics.

The surgeon does a final check to make sure the lens is in good position. The wound is tested to ensure that it is watertight, and the lid supporting speculum is removed. Immediately following the treatment, the patient is monitored in the postoperative holding area and finally discharged.

Chapter Nine

What Happens after Your Cataract Treatment?

The postoperative period involves the instillation of drops for a few weeks while the eye heals. The medications that are applied include antibiotics and anti-inflammatory agents. The anti-inflammatory drugs may be steroids or nonsteroidal anti-inflammatory agents (chemically similar to aspirin formulated as a drop). Recently, the trend has been to use both types of anti-inflammatory agents, as each type of drug acts through a slightly different pathway. You will be provided with a medication schedule, and a list of activities to avoid.

I do ask that patients take a one to two week hiatus from swimming, hot tubs or other activities that could put their eyes in contact with "common" water. Pools, hot tubs and other forms of common water often serve as breeding grounds for microbes (otherwise referred to by my eight year-old son, Alexander, as "tiny, ugly germs!") which may infect an incompletely-healed surgical wound. Typically patients resume most of their normal activity level within a few days, as small-incision surgery has largely eliminated the need for an extended convalescence.

Patients are seen on the day after their procedure, and usually are fully rehabilitated within a month of their treatment.
Congratulations! It is time to enjoy your new and improved vision!

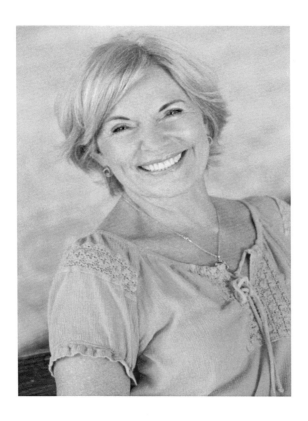

Figure 7   A very happy patient, after cataract surgery.

Chapter Ten

Laser Vision Correction

Advances in cataract surgery have made significant inroads into the refractive surgery arena, but for more than a decade LASIK has been king. **LASIK** is an eponym for the term **Laser-As**sisted in-situ **K**eratomileusis. Unlike cataract surgery, LASIK, and all forms of laser vision correction, improve the eye's ability to focus by changing the contour of the cornea.

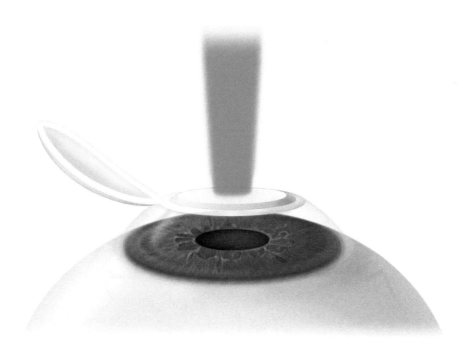

Figure 8   Laser-Assisted in-situ Keratomileusis (LASIK)

Accordingly, the laser vision correction (LVC) procedures fall under the category of **keratorefractive** ("cornea focusing") surgery.

Photorefractive Keratectomy (PRK) is the other form of laser vision correction.

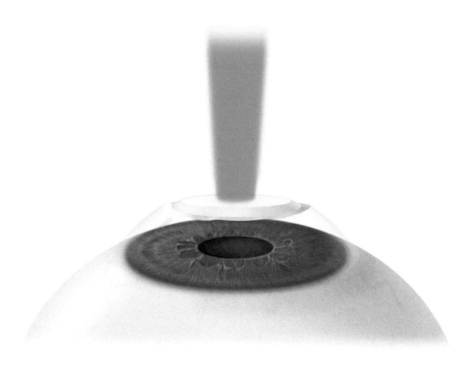

Picture Courtesy of American Academy of Ophthalmology

Figure 9 Photorefractive Keratectomy (PRK)

At the time of this writing, most forms of laser correction require the use of one type of laser, the **excimer** laser. The name excimer is derived from the term <u>exc</u>ited d<u>imer</u>, which generates the 193 nanometer wavelength laser beam (again, a cocktail party point that has the potential to give you that lonely feeling). The significance of the laser wavelength is important on at least two levels. First, the 193nm beam does not pass beyond the cornea, and so, there is no risk of the laser affecting the sensitive intraocular tissues. Secondly, the laser does not create a "collateral thermal effect," that is, the only tissue that is affected by the laser is the tissue which the laser actually lands upon. The adjacent corneal tissue is totally unchanged (otherwise, heat conducted to the adjacent corneal tissue would cause a secondary, unpredictable visual effect).

A basic understanding of corneal anatomy is helpful in understanding how the LVC treatments work. The cornea is the outer "window" and first refractive surface of the eye (Figure 10).

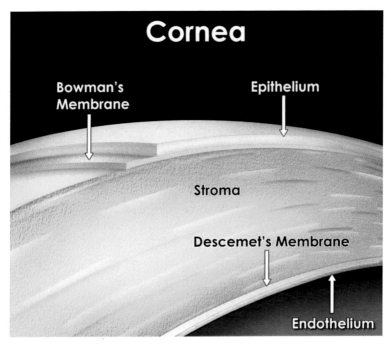

Figure 10 Layers of the Cornea

The cornea consists of three primary layers. The first is the outer **epithelium,** which is comprised of 6-7 layers of cells which are able to regenerate rapidly. The epithelium rests upon **Bowman's Membrane,** which defines the very front of the middle corneal layer known as the **stroma**. Unlike the epithelium, the stroma has relatively few cells and is composed primarily of protein. The stroma makes up approximately 85% of the corneal thickness, and compared to the epithelial layer, the stroma has very limited ability to regenerate. The third layer of the cornea is the **endothelial cell layer**. This is the innermost layer of cells which act as the cornea's internal "pump." The endothelial cells work constantly to try to maintain the cornea in a relatively dehydrated state, which keeps the cornea crystal clear. The endothelial cells are arranged as a single cell layer. There is essentially no regeneration of these cells, so when they are lost, the remaining endothelial cells must be able to compensate for this loss or the cornea swells, resulting in decreased vision. Corneal swelling (edema) from endothelial cell loss can be treated by one of the corneal transplantation techniques: **penetrating keratoplasty** or **Descemet's Stripping Automated Endothelial Keratoplasty** (DSAEK).

Laser vision correction improves vision by subtly altering the curvature of the cornea. There are currently only two mechanisms available to change the cornea via laser. The first method works via the application of **excimer laser** energy directly to the surface of the cornea, and the second method involves the use of the laser energy just under the surface of the cornea after a thin, hinged flap is created.

Listed below are the names and abbreviations of frequently performed surface treatments.

- Photorefractive keratectomy – PRK (Figure 9)
- ASA – Advanced Surface Ablation
- LASEK – Laser-assisted epithelial keratomileusis
- Epi – LASEK – (same as LASEK)

The list above represents different surgeons' approaches as to how they manage the eye prior to and immediately after the laser application. The four procedures listed above all have in common the direct application of the excimer laser to the surface of the cornea. Considering the commonalities these techniques share, it is not surprising to learn that the outcomes of these procedures are essentially identical.

LASIK has a more limited subgroup of monikers. The following is a list of these variations and the accompanying definitions.

- LASIK –(*Laser-assisted in situ keratomileusis*). A bladed instrument called a **microkeratome** is used to create the superficial corneal flap. These instruments have essentially two components: the *base* is a suction ring which engages the eye, and the *head*, which consists of a gear or piston-driven apparatus which supports a guarded, oscillating blade. The flap is created as the head translates across the eye which is being held by the suction mechanism on the base.

- All-Laser LASIK or "No-Blade" LASIK. The concept of this variation is that the superficial flap is created with a highly accurate **femtosecond** laser. The process is more controlled than bladed LASIK as the surgeon is able to "customize" such factors as flap thickness, hinge position and flap diameter. The flap is reflected and the corrective treatment is achieved by subsequently applying the excimer laser. (Figure 8) Therefore (as of press time), two lasers are required to perform true "blade free" LASIK.

But beware! There are still a few "questionable" marketing practices, advertising their surface treatment as being "blade free laser correction." It is important to verify that you are actually getting blade free LASIK! When in doubt, speak to the surgeon directly. Any surgeon is happy to have their patient at ease with the procedure (and actually bringing you into the laser treatment room to show you the two lasers is a great way to "desensitize" patients to the anxiety of treatment day).

- Sub-Bowman's Keratomileusis (SBK) . An "all laser" procedure that depends upon the extreme accuracy of the femtosecond laser to create an ultra-thin flap just beneath Bowman's Membrane.

Chapter 11

Other Surgical Methods for Vision Correction

The use of **implantable contact lenses** (ICL) (Figure 11) has met with some level of popularity in Europe. The ICL has found its greatest use in eyes that are not candidates for laser vision correction.

Similar to cataract surgery, a small incision is made in the peripheral cornea and a synthetic intraocular lens is placed in the eye without removing the eye's natural crystalline lens.

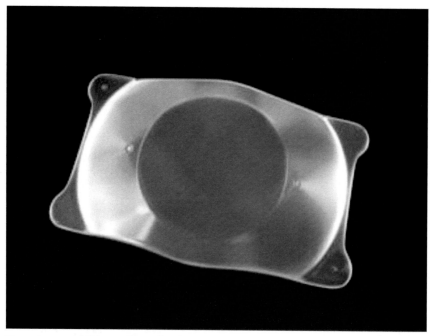

Courtesy of Staar Surgical

Figure 11 Implantable Contact Lens (ICL)

The ICL is a reasonable alternative for patients who have thin corneas or whose degree of nearsightedness is extremely high.

INTACS were approved for the treatment of relatively low degrees of nearsightedness in the 1990s. INTACs are semi-circular implants that are placed within the stroma of the cornea; hence they are classified as intracorneal ring segments. The segments are placed in the mid-periphery of the cornea and improve the uncorrected vision in myopes by flattening the central cornea. While intracorneal ring segments were effective for low degrees of myopia, laser vision correction was at least as effective as INTACs, and could be performed without incurring the cost of an implant.

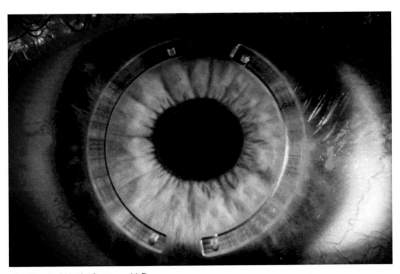

Courtesy of Mario Serrano, M.D.

Figure 12   Intracorneal ring segments, (INTACs)

The intense competition in the vision correction market prevented INTACS from gaining any significant market share; however, the intracorneal implant has found a niche market by being a popular and effective treatment in the treatment of a corneal condition called **keratoconus**.

Conclusion

Your eyes allow you to navigate through your world seamlessly. Whether your goal is to be able to see well enough to pilot an airplane, target shoot, or merely feel more confident when driving, your vision can be customized in order to meet your needs. The process of personalizing cataract surgery has evolved through the decades and is now available in a day-stay setting under local anesthesia. Today's cataract procedures offer patients a previously unattainable level of independent visual function, from the flexibility offered by the presbyopic implants to the clarity of astigmatism-free sight.

Likewise, laser vision correction has made tremendous strides since it's advent in the 1990s. The accuracy and safety of today's "custom" and "no-blade" technologies have resulted in unprecedented outcomes while minimizing risk. Hopefully, the terms and concepts described in this book will give you the insight to choose the procedure that fits your needs and thereby helps you realize an enhanced level of visual performance and enjoyment.